ULTIMATE

Music Trivia
for Adults

Leon Simonds

Share Your Musical Journey!

If our trivia book has added a note of joy to your day, consider sharing your thoughts on Amazon. Your insights not only help fellow music lovers find their next read but also support us in composing future editions. Reviews are a way to connect with others in the community and express what resonated with you.

Take a moment to leave a review and let's spread the harmony!

TABLE OF CONTENTS

INTRODUCTION

Welcome to the ultimate journey through the rhythms and beats of history with our music trivia book, designed exclusively for adults who cherish the harmonies and stories behind the songs. Whether you're a casual listener or a dedicated audiophile, this book offers a symphony of 150 questions that will challenge your musical knowledge and provide a delightful encore of entertainment.

Each page presents three carefully curated questions, ranging from classical compositions to modern-day chart-toppers, ensuring a diverse medley of genres and eras. Turn the page, and you'll find not only the answers but also a concerto of amusing anecdotes, fascinating facts, and light-hearted explanations that will resonate with music lovers of all backgrounds.

So, tune your curiosity, sharpen your wits, and prepare to embark on an auditory adventure that celebrates the vast and vibrant world of music. Let the trivia begin!

MASTERING THE GAME

Welcome to the next stage of your musical quest! This chapter is your backstage pass to mastering the art of playing our music trivia book. Here's how to make the most of your experience and enjoy every note of this melodious challenge.

Setting the Stage

Before diving into the questions, find a comfortable spot where you can relax and immerse yourself in the music world. Whether it's a cozy armchair or a sunny spot in the park, make sure it's a place where you can concentrate and enjoy the game without interruptions.

Solo or Ensemble

Decide if you're going on a solo tour or forming a band. You can play by yourself, testing your own knowledge, or turn it into a social event by challenging friends and family. If you're playing in a group, consider taking turns reading the questions aloud and keeping score to see who has the most musical prowess.

The Rhythm of the Game

Start by reading each question carefully and pondering your answer. Don't rush—treat it like you're savoring a fine symphony. Once you've made your choice, flip to the answers page to see if you hit the right note.

MASTERING THE GAME

Learning the Melodies
Each answer comes with a short, fun explanation or fact from the music world. Take the time to read these tidbits—they're designed to entertain and educate, adding depth to your understanding of music history and culture.

Keeping Score
If you're feeling competitive, keep track of your correct answers. Set a goal for yourself or your group, and see if you can surpass it. Celebrate your victories with a favorite tune or a dance break!

Encore!
Don't stop at the end of the book. Use it as a stepping stone to explore more about the artists, genres, and historical moments you've encountered. Our trivia is just the beginning of your musical exploration.

Remember, the key to enjoying this trivia book is not just in getting the answers right, but in appreciating the rich tapestry of stories and sounds that make up the world of music. So tune in, play on, and let the good times roll!

Question 1: Which artist is known as the "King of Pop"?

(A)	Elvis Presley	(B)	Michael Jackson
(C)	Prince	(D)	Justin Bieber

Question 2: Who composed the famous four-note motif in the Symphony No. 5?

(A)	Wolfgang Amadeus Mozart	(B)	Johann Sebastian Bach
(C)	Ludwig van Beethoven	(D)	Franz Schubert

Question 3: What is the best-selling single of all time?

(A)	"Candle in the Wind"	(B)	"I Will Always Love You"
(C)	"Happy"	(D)	"Despacito"

Question 1
B) Michael Jackson

Michael Jackson is globally recognized as the "King of Pop" for his groundbreaking contributions to music, dance, and fashion, along with his publicized personal life. His 1982 album "Thriller" is the best-selling album of all time.

Question 2
C) Ludwig van Beethoven

Beethoven's Symphony No. 5 is famous for its short-short-short-long motif, often interpreted as "fate knocking at the door." This motif opens the first movement and is one of the most recognized in classical music history.

Question 3
A) "Candle in the Wind"

Elton John's "Candle in the Wind 1997," a tribute to Diana, Princess of Wales, is the best-selling single since charts began, with 33 million copies sold. However, Bing Crosby's "White Christmas" holds the all-time record with estimated sales of over 50 million copies.

Question 4: Which band released the hit song "Bohemian Rhapsody"?

A. The Beatles

B. Queen

C. Led Zeppelin

D. Pink Floyd

Question 5: Which instrument did Miles Davis famously play?

A. Trumpet

B. Saxophone

C. Piano

D. Drums

Question 6: What genre is Taylor Swift most associated with?

A. Pop

B. Country

C. Rock

D. R&B

Question 4
B) Queen

"Bohemian Rhapsody" is a song by the English rock band Queen. It was written by Freddie Mercury for the band's 1975 album "A Night at the Opera." The song has no chorus, instead consisting of several sections: a ballad segment, an operatic passage, a hard rock part, and a reflective coda.

Question 5
A) Trumpet

Miles Davis was an American jazz trumpeter, bandleader, and composer. He is among the most influential and acclaimed figures in the history of jazz and 20th-century music. Davis was known for his lyrical, introspective trumpet playing and was at the forefront of several major developments in jazz music.

Question 6
A) Pop

Taylor Swift is most associated with the pop genre, especially after her transition from country music with her album "1989" in 2014. She has since explored various styles, including synth-pop, indie folk, and alternative.

Question 7: Who is the composer of the "Moonlight Sonata"?

A. Claude Debussy

B. Franz Liszt

C. Ludwig van Beethoven

D. Frédéric Chopin

Question 8: Which song features the lyrics "Just a small town girl, living in a lonely world"?

A. "Sweet Child O' Mine"

B. "Stairway to Heaven"

C. "Don't Stop Believin'"

D. "Hotel California"

Question 9: Which artist released the album "Thriller" in 1982?

A. Madonna

B. Michael Jackson

C. Prince

D. David Bowie

Question 7
C) Ludwig van Beethoven

Beethoven composed the "Moonlight Sonata" (Piano Sonata No. 14 in C-sharp minor, "Quasi una fantasia", Op. 27, No. 2). The piece, completed in 1801 and published in 1802, is admired for its serene and dreamy first movement.

Question 8
C) "Don't Stop Believin'"

The lyrics "Just a small town girl, living in a lonely world" are from the song "Don't Stop Believin'" by the band Journey. Released in 1981, it became a top hit and has since been a popular anthem featured in many movies and TV shows.

Question 9
B) Michael Jackson

Michael Jackson released the album "Thriller" on November 29, 1982. It became the best-selling album of all time, with hits like "Billie Jean" and "Beat It," and showcased Jackson's ability to blend pop, rock, and R&B.

Question 10: Who is the lead singer of the band U2?

A. Bono

B. Mick Jagger

C. Bruce Springsteen

D. Jon Bon Jovi

Question 11: Which classical composer became deaf later in life?

A. Antonio Vivaldi

B. Johann Sebastian Bach

C. Ludwig van Beethoven

D. Wolfgang Amadeus Mozart

Question 12: Which song famously begins with the line "Is this the real life? Is this just fantasy?"

A. "Imagine"

B. "Bohemian Rhapsody"

C. "Like a Rolling Stone"

D. "Hotel California"

Question 10
A) Bono

Bono, born Paul David Hewson, is the lead singer of the Irish rock band U2. Known for his distinctive voice and passionate performances, he has been a key figure in U2's success and is also recognized for his activism.

Question 11
C) Ludwig van Beethoven

Beethoven, one of the most famous classical composers, experienced progressive hearing loss beginning in his mid-20s and was almost completely deaf by his mid-40s. Despite his deafness, he continued to compose masterpieces, including the Ninth Symphony.

Question 12
B) "Bohemian Rhapsody"

The song "Bohemian Rhapsody" by Queen begins with the lines "Is this the real life? Is this just fantasy?" It's known for its unique structure, blending rock, ballad, and opera styles, and remains one of the band's most iconic songs.

Question 13: Which artist is known for the hit "Purple Rain"?

A	Bruce Springsteen	B	Prince
C	David Bowie	D	Elton John

Question 14: What year did The Beatles release their first single?

A	1960	B	1962
C	1964	D	1966

Question 15: Which artist is known for the hit song "Firework"?

A	Katy Perry	B	Lady Gaga
C	Adele	D	Rihanna

Question 13
B) Prince

Prince is known for the hit "Purple Rain," which is a song by Prince and the Revolution from the 1984 album of the same name. It is considered one of Prince's signature songs and has been widely acclaimed for its mix of rock, R&B, gospel, and orchestral music.

Question 14
B) 1962

The Beatles released their first single, "Love Me Do," in the United Kingdom on *October 5, 1962*. This marked the beginning of what would become a monumental career in music history, leading to the phenomenon known as "Beatlemania."

Question 15
A) Katy Perry

"Firework" is a hit song by Katy Perry, released in 2010 as part of her album "Teenage Dream." The song is known for its empowering message and catchy chorus, becoming an anthem for self-confidence and celebration of individuality.

Question 16: Who won the first ever Grammy for Best Rap Performance?

A	DJ Jazzy Jeff & The Fresh Prince	B	LL Cool J
C	Salt-N-Pepa	D	Run-D.M.C.

Question 17: What is the name of the famous British rock band formed in London in 1968?

A	Pink Floyd	B	The Rolling Stones
C	Led Zeppelin	D	The Who

QQueen was inducted into the Grammy Hall of Fame in 2009?

A	We Will Rock You	B	Bohemian Rhapsody
C	Another One Bites the Dust	D	Radio Ga Ga

Question 16
A) DJ Jazzy Jeff & The Fresh Prince

DJ Jazzy Jeff & The Fresh Prince won the first Grammy for Best Rap Performance in 1989 for their hit "Parents Just Don't Understand." This was a significant moment as it marked the recognition of rap by the mainstream music industry.

Question 17
C) Led Zeppelin

Led Zeppelin, formed in London in 1968, is renowned for their influential role in the development of rock music. With hits like "Stairway to Heaven" and "Whole Lotta Love," they are considered one of the pioneering bands of heavy metal and hard rock genres.

Question 18
B) Bohemian Rhapsody

"Bohemian Rhapsody" by Queen was inducted into the Grammy Hall of Fame in 2009. This iconic song, released in 1975, is known for its unique structure and has remained a staple in rock music history.

Question 19: Which artist's real name is Stefani Joanne Angelina Germanotta?

A. Sia

B. Madonna

C. Lady Gaga

D. Pink

Question 20: What was the first video ever played on MTV?

A. Video Killed the Radio Star

B. Thriller

C. Money for Nothing

D. Sledgehammer

Question 21: Which composer is known for the "Four Seasons" concertos?

A. Johann Sebastian Bach

B. Wolfgang Amadeus Mozart

C. Antonio Vivaldi

D. Ludwig van Beethoven

Question 19
C) Lady Gaga

Stefani Joanne Angelina Germanotta is better known by her stage name, Lady Gaga. She is an American singer, songwriter, and actress known for her image reinventions and musical versatility.

Question 20
A) Video Killed the Radio Star

"Video Killed the Radio Star" by The Buggles was the first video ever played on MTV when it launched on August 1, 1981. The song's theme was a commentary on the impact of modern technology on media.

Question 21
C) Antonio Vivaldi

Antonio Vivaldi, an Italian Baroque composer, is famous for his violin concertos known as "The Four Seasons." These four concertos each represent a different season and are some of the most popular pieces in the classical music repertoire.

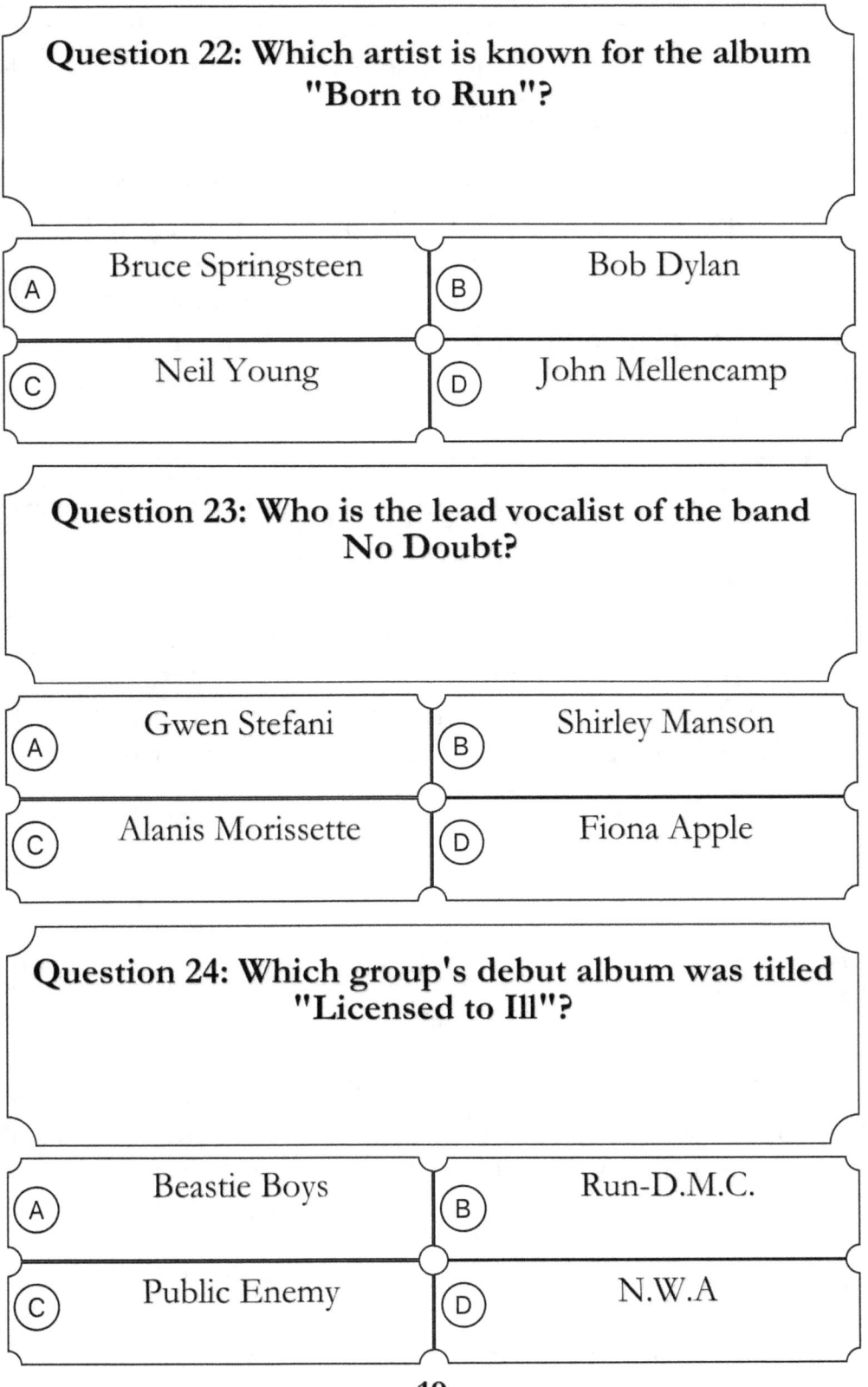

Question 22: Which artist is known for the album "Born to Run"?

A	Bruce Springsteen	B	Bob Dylan
C	Neil Young	D	John Mellencamp

Question 23: Who is the lead vocalist of the band No Doubt?

A	Gwen Stefani	B	Shirley Manson
C	Alanis Morissette	D	Fiona Apple

Question 24: Which group's debut album was titled "Licensed to Ill"?

A	Beastie Boys	B	Run-D.M.C.
C	Public Enemy	D	N.W.A

Question 22
A) Bruce Springsteen

Bruce Springsteen is renowned for his album "Born to Run," released in 1975. The album became a commercial success and is celebrated for its rich storytelling and energetic rock anthems, encapsulating the essence of American life.

Question 23
A) Gwen Stefani

Gwen Stefani is the lead vocalist of the band No Doubt. The band gained mainstream success in the 1990s with their ska-punk influenced sound, and Stefani's distinctive voice played a significant role in their popularity.

Question 24
A) Beastie Boys

The Beastie Boys released their debut album "Licensed to Ill" in 1986. It was the first rap LP to top the Billboard album chart, and its success helped bring hip-hop to a wider audience.

Question 25: Which musician is nicknamed "The Boss"?

A. Jon Bon Jovi

B. Bruce Springsteen

C. Bob Dylan

D. Tom Petty

Question 26: What is the highest-selling album of the 21st century?

A. 21 by Adele

B. The Eminem Show by Eminem

C. Hybrid Theory by Linkin Park

D. Confessions by Usher

Question 27: Who composed the opera "The Magic Flute"?

A. Richard Wagner

B. Giuseppe Verdi

C. Gioachino Rossini

D. Wolfgang Amadeus Mozart

Question 25
B) Bruce Springsteen

Bruce Springsteen has long been referred to as "The Boss," a nickname that reflects his commanding presence and leadership in live performances, as well as his working-class advocacy in his music. His career spans several decades, with numerous hits and accolades.

Question 26
A) 21 by Adele

Adele's album "21" has achieved significant commercial success, becoming the highest-selling album of the 21st century. It features hits like "Rolling in the Deep" and "Someone Like You," and has won numerous awards, including the Grammy for Album of the Year.

Question 27
D) Wolfgang Amadeus Mozart

"The Magic Flute" is one of Mozart's most famous operas, known for its beautiful arias and complex characters. It premiered in 1791, just months before the composer's death, and has since become a staple in the opera repertoire.

Question 28: Which band's lead singer is Thom Yorke?

A   Radiohead

B   Coldplay

C   Oasis

D   Blur

Question 29: Who is credited with inventing the solid-body electric guitar?

A   Les Paul

B   Leo Fender

C   Jimi Hendrix

D   Chuck Berry

Question 30: Which iconic song begins with the line "Mama, just killed a man"?

A   Stairway to Heaven

B   Hotel California

C   Sweet Child O' Mine

D   Bohemian Rhapsody

Question 28
A) Radiohead

Thom Yorke is the lead singer of the English rock band Radiohead, known for their experimental approach to music and their influential albums such as "OK Computer" and "Kid A." Yorke's distinctive voice and the band's innovative sound have garnered critical acclaim worldwide.

Question 29
A) Les Paul.

Les Paul is widely recognized for his contributions to the development of the solid-body electric guitar, which made the sound of rock and roll possible. His innovative designs and techniques transformed the music industry and influenced countless musicians.

Question 30
D) Bohemian Rhapsody.

The opening line "Mama, just killed a man" is from Queen's epic song "Bohemian Rhapsody." Released in 1975, it's known for its unique structure, blending rock, balladry, opera, and classical music, becoming one of the band's signature songs and a classic of rock music.

Question 31: What's the name of the dance craze Michael Jackson popularized?

A	The Twist	B	The Moonwalk
C	The Macarena	D	Gangnam Style

Question 32: Which artist's debut album is titled "The Fame"?

A	Adele	B	Lady Gaga
C	Katy Perry	D	Rihanna

Question 33: Which band's album is called "Dark Side of the Moon"?

A	The Beatles	B	Pink Floyd
C	Led Zeppelin	D	The Rolling Stones

Question 31
B) The Moonwalk.

Michael Jackson famously performed the Moonwalk for the first time on television during the Motown 25: Yesterday, Today, Forever special in 1983. This dance move, which creates the illusion of gliding backwards, became his signature move and is still associated with him today.

Question 32
B) Lady Gaga.

Lady Gaga's debut album, "The Fame," was released in 2008 and included hits like "Just Dance" and "Poker Face." The album's themes revolve around fame, love, and wealth, and it played a significant role in propelling her to stardom.

Question 33
B) Pink Floyd.

"Dark Side of the Moon," released in 1973, is one of Pink Floyd's most acclaimed albums. Known for its progressive rock sound and thematic exploration of conflict, greed, time, and mental illness, it's one of the best-selling albums worldwide.

Question 34: Which singer is known as "The Material Girl"?

A	Madonna	B	Cher
C	Beyonc?	D	Britney Spears

Question 35: What's the name of the famous club where The Beatles played before their rise to fame?

A	The Troubadour	B	The Viper Room
C	The Cavern Club	D	CBGB

Question 36: Which song by The Police starts with "Every breath you take"?

A	Roxanne	B	Message in a Bottle
C	Every Breath You Take	D	Walking on the Moon

Question 34
A) Madonna.

Madonna is often referred to as "The Material Girl," a nickname that originated from her hit song with the same title. The song's popularity and its reflection of Madonna's persona in the 1980s helped cement this moniker in pop culture.

Question 35
C) The Cavern Club.

The Cavern Club in Liverpool is where The Beatles performed during their early years, helping to establish their popularity before they became international superstars. The club has since become a landmark and a symbol of the band's beginnings.

Question 36
C) Every Breath You Take.

"Every Breath You Take" is a song by The Police from their 1983 album "Synchronicity." Written by Sting, the song is known for its haunting melody and lyrics that can be interpreted as both a love song and a tale of obsession. It became one of their biggest hits.

Question 37: Which artist is known for the hit single "Hello"?

A	Adele	B	Beyonc?
C	Sam Smith	D	Ed Sheeran

Question 38: What instrument is Robert Smith of The Cure known for playing?

A	Drums	B	Guitar
C	Bass	D	Keyboard

Question 39: Which group is known for the hit "Waterloo"?

A	ABBA	B	The Beatles
C	Queen	D	Fleetwood Mac

Question 37
A) Adele.

Adele's "Hello" was the lead single from her third studio album, "25," released in 2015. The song achieved widespread acclaim and commercial success, topping charts around the world and becoming one of her signature songs.

Question 38
B) Guitar.

Robert Smith, the lead vocalist and guitarist of The Cure, is particularly known for his distinctive guitar playing style. His use of chorus and flanger effects has been influential in the post-punk and new wave genres. The Cure's sound is often characterized by his melodic guitar lines.

Question 39
A) ABBA.

ABBA, the Swedish pop group, won the Eurovision Song Contest in 1974 with "Waterloo," which became an international hit and launched their career. The song is celebrated for its catchy tune and historical references.

Question 40: Who composed the iconic film score for "Star Wars"?

A. Hans Zimmer

B. John Williams

C. Danny Elfman

D. Howard Shore

Question 41: Which artist is known for the anthem "Born in the U.S.A."?

A. Bruce Springsteen

B. Bob Dylan

C. John Mellencamp

D. Tom Petty

Question 42: Which band's album "Rumours" won the Grammy for Album of the Year in 1978?

A. The Eagles

B. Pink Floyd

C. Fleetwood Mac

D. The Rolling Stones

Question 40
B) John Williams.

John Williams is the acclaimed composer behind the "Star Wars" soundtrack, known for its memorable themes that have become synonymous with the franchise. His work has helped define the sound of modern cinema.

Question 41
A) Bruce Springsteen.

"Born in the U.S.A." is one of Bruce Springsteen's most famous songs, released on the album of the same name in 1984. The song is often misinterpreted as purely patriotic, but it actually discusses the challenges faced by Vietnam veterans returning to America.

Question 42
C) Fleetwood Mac.

Fleetwood Mac's "Rumours" is one of the best-selling albums of all time and won the Grammy for Album of the Year in 1978. The album's production was marked by personal turmoil among band members, which influenced its emotional depth.

Question 43: What's the title of Elton John's tribute to Marilyn Monroe?

A. Candle in the Wind

B. Rocket Man

C. Tiny Dancer

D. Your Song

Question 44: Which artist is known for the hit "I Will Always Love You"?

A. Mariah Carey

B. Whitney Houston

C. Celine Dion

D. Adele

Question 45: Which band is known for the anthem "Smells Like Teen Spirit"?

A. Nirvana

B. Metallica

C. Green Day

D. Red Hot Chili Peppers

Question 43
A) Candle in the Wind.

"Candle in the Wind" was originally written in 1973 as a tribute to Marilyn Monroe. Elton John later re-recorded the song in 1997 as a tribute to Princess Diana, with the new version becoming the fastest-selling single in UK chart history.

Question 44
B) Whitney Houston.

"I Will Always Love You" was famously covered by Whitney Houston for the soundtrack of the film "The Bodyguard" in 1992. Her powerful rendition became one of the best-selling singles of all time. The song was originally written and recorded by Dolly Parton in 1973.

Question 45
A) Nirvana.

"Smells Like Teen Spirit" is a song by the American rock band Nirvana. It is the opening track and lead single from their second album, "Nevermind" (1991), and is often hailed as an anthem of Generation X. The song's unexpected success propelled Nirvana to the forefront of the grunge movement.

Question 46: Which artist released the album "Back to Black" in 2006?

A	Amy Winehouse	B	Adele
C	Lana Del Rey	D	Duffy

Question 47: Which composer is known for the "Brandenburg Concertos"?

A	Wolfgang Amadeus Mozart	B	Ludwig van Beethoven
C	Johann Sebastian Bach	D	Antonio Vivaldi

Question 48: Which artist is known for the song "Ring of Fire"?

A	Johnny Cash	B	Elvis Presley
C	Bob Dylan	D	Willie Nelson

Question 46
A) Amy Winehouse.

"Back to Black" is the second and final studio album by English singer Amy Winehouse. It was released in October 2006 and features the hit singles "Rehab" and "Back to Black." The album received critical acclaim and won five Grammy Awards, including Best Pop Vocal Album.

Question 47
C) Johann Sebastian Bach.

The "Brandenburg Concertos" are a collection of six instrumental works composed by Johann Sebastian Bach. They are considered some of the finest orchestral compositions of the Baroque era and showcase Bach's ability to blend Italian and German musical styles.

Question 48
A) Johnny Cash.

"Ring of Fire" is one of Johnny Cash's most famous songs. It was co-written by June Carter Cash and Merle Kilgore and became a hit in 1963. The song is known for its mariachi-style horn arrangement and its place in country music history.

Question 49: Who is the lead singer of the band Radiohead?

A. Chris Martin

B. Thom Yorke

C. Damon Albarn

D. Bono

Question 50: Which artist is known for the hit "Take On Me"?

A. a-ha

B. Duran Duran

C. Wham!

D. Depeche Mode

Question 51: Which composer is famed for the "Bol?ro"?

A. Igor Stravinsky

B. Maurice Ravel

C. George Gershwin

D. Sergei Rachmaninoff

Question 49
B) Thom Yorke.

Thom Yorke is the lead vocalist and primary songwriter of the English rock band Radiohead. Known for his distinctive voice and experimental approach to music, Yorke has been a pivotal figure in the band's success since its formation in the 1980s. Radiohead's work is highly regarded for its innovation and depth.

Question 50
A) a-ha.

"Take On Me" is a song by the Norwegian synth-pop band a-ha, released in 1985. The song became a global hit, and its innovative music video, featuring a mix of live-action and pencil-sketch animation, won six awards at the 1986 MTV Video Music Awards.

Question 51
B) Maurice Ravel.

Maurice Ravel's "Bol?ro" is known for its repetitive melody and increasingly loud dynamics. Composed in 1928, it's one of his most famous works, originally written as a ballet commissioned by Russian ballerina Ida Rubinstein. The piece has been used in many films and figure skating routines.

Question 52: Which band's debut album is "Appetite for Destruction"?

A	Guns N' Roses	B	Metallica
C	AC/DC	D	Nirvana

Question 53: Which artist is known for the song "Hallelujah"?

A	Leonard Cohen	B	Jeff Buckley
C	Rufus Wainwright	D	John Cale

Question 54: Which artist is known for the song "Like a Rolling Stone"?

A	Bob Dylan	B	Bruce Springsteen
C	Neil Young	D	Tom Petty

Question 52
A) Guns N' Roses.

"Appetite for Destruction" is the debut studio album by American hard rock band Guns N' Roses, released in 1987. It's known for hits like "Welcome to the Jungle" and "Sweet Child o' Mine," and it became a massive commercial success, shaping the band's career.

Question 53
A) Leonard Cohen.

Leonard Cohen originally wrote and recorded "Hallelujah," which appeared on his 1984 album "Various Positions." The song has since been covered by many artists, but Cohen's version remains the definitive one, known for its emotional depth and lyrical complexity. Jeff Buckley's cover is also widely acclaimed.

Question 54
A) Bob Dylan.

"Like a Rolling Stone" is a song by American singer-songwriter Bob Dylan. Released as a single in 1965, it's considered one of the most influential compositions in postwar popular music and marked a departure from Dylan's earlier folk music style.

Question 55: Which artist is widely known as the "Queen of Soul"?

A. Aretha Franklin

B. Whitney Houston

C. Diana Ross

D. Tina Turner

Question 56: Which band is known for the album "Nevermind"?

A. Nirvana

B. Metallica

C. Red Hot Chili Peppers

D. Pearl Jam

Question 57: What's the name of the singer known as "The Voice"?

A. Frank Sinatra

B. Elvis Presley

C. Michael Bubl?

D. Whitney Houston

Question 55
A) Aretha Franklin

Aretha Franklin is widely known as the "Queen of Soul" for her powerful voice and impactful songs that defined a generation. Her hits like "Respect" and "Chain of Fools" have become anthems of empowerment and soul music staples. Franklin's influence on the genre and her numerous awards, including 18 Grammys, solidify her royal status in music history.

Question 56
A) Nirvana

Nirvana's second studio album, "Nevermind," released in 1991, is one of the most influential albums of all time. It brought the grunge genre to the mainstream, largely thanks to the hit song "Smells Like Teen Spirit." The album's success marked a shift in music and has since been certified Diamond in the US.

Question 57
A) Frank Sinatra

Frank Sinatra earned the nickname "The Voice" for his impeccable vocal control and ability to convey emotion through his singing. His smooth, crooning style made him one of the most popular and influential musical artists of the 20th century, with timeless hits like "Fly Me to the Moon" and "My Way."

Question 58: Which artist is known for the hit "Heart of Glass"?

A. Madonna

B. Cyndi Lauper

C. Blondie

D. Pat Benatar

Question 59: Which group released the song "Hotel California"?

A. The Eagles

B. Fleetwood Mac

C. The Rolling Stones

D. Pink Floyd

Question 60: Who composed the "Rite of Spring"?

A. Igor Stravinsky

B. Ludwig van Beethoven

C. Johann Sebastian Bach

D. Pyotr Ilyich Tchaikovsky

Question 58
C) Blondie

"Heart of Glass" is a song by the American rock band Blondie, written by singer Debbie Harry and guitarist Chris Stein. Released in 1979, it was a major success, reaching the top of the charts in several countries and is one of the band's signature songs. Its innovative disco-rock sound was influential in the new wave genre.

Question 59
A) The Eagles

"Hotel California" is a classic hit by The Eagles, featured on their 1976 album of the same name. The song is known for its distinctive guitar solo and cryptic lyrics, which have led to much speculation about their meaning. It remains one of the band's most famous and enduring songs.

Question 60
A) Igor Stravinsky

Igor Stravinsky composed "The Rite of Spring" in 1913. This avant-garde piece is famous for its revolutionary approach to rhythm and dissonance, which caused a stir at its premiere, leading to one of the most notorious riots in music history. It's now considered one of the most influential works of the 20th century.

Question 61: Who is the "Prince of Motown"?

A	Marvin Gaye	B	Stevie Wonder
C	Smokey Robinson	D	Lionel Richie

Question 62: Which artist is called "The Boss"?

A	Bruce Springsteen	B	Jon Bon Jovi
C	Billy Joel	D	Bob Dylan

Question 63: Which song is famously known as "The Anthem of the Counterculture"?

A	Imagine	B	Blowin' in the Wind
C	Give Peace a Chance	D	Fortunate Son

Question 61
C) Smokey Robinson

Smokey Robinson earned the title "Prince of Motown" for his contributions to the Motown record label, both as a performer and as a songwriter. He helped define the label's sound with hits like "Tears of a Clown" and "Tracks of My Tears," and his smooth voice and emotive lyrics have made him a soul music legend.

Question 62
A) Bruce Springsteen

Bruce Springsteen is affectionately known as "The Boss," a nickname that reflects his commanding presence and leadership in live performances. He is renowned for his work with the E Street Band, his poetic lyrics, and his marathon concerts. His music, including hits like "Born to Run," has resonated with fans for decades.

Question 63
B) Blowin' in the Wind

"Blowin' in the Wind" by Bob Dylan became an anthem for the 1960s counterculture, civil rights, and anti-war movements. Its poignant lyrics pose rhetorical questions about peace, war, and freedom, which resonated deeply with the sentiments of the era's youth and activists. Dylan's songwriting prowess is showcased in this timeless classic.

Question 64: What's the title of the song with the lyric "I see a little silhouetto of a man"?

A	Rocket Man	B	Stairway to Heaven
C	Bohemian Rhapsody	D	Hotel California

Question 65: Which artist is known for "The Times They Are a-Changin'"?

A	Bob Dylan	B	Neil Young
C	Joni Mitchell	D	Bruce Springsteen

Question 66: Who is known as the "Godfather of Punk"?

A	Iggy Pop	B	Joey Ramone
C	Patti Smith	D	Johnny Rotten

Question 64
C) Bohemian Rhapsody

The lyric is from Queen's "Bohemian Rhapsody," a song known for its complex structure, mixing rock, ballad, and opera styles. Released in 1975, it became one of the band's greatest hits and is celebrated for its innovative approach and Freddie Mercury's powerful vocals.

Question 65
A) Bob Dylan

"The Times They Are a-Changin'" is a song written by Bob Dylan and released as the title track of his 1964 album. The song captures the spirit of social and political upheaval that characterized the 1960s. Dylan's poignant lyrics and folk music style made this song an anthem for change and a testament to his influence as a songwriter and musician.

Question 66
A) Iggy Pop

Iggy Pop, lead singer of The Stooges, is often referred to as the "Godfather of Punk" for his influential role in the early punk rock movement. His wild stage antics and raw sound helped set the stage for many punk bands that followed. Iggy's music and persona embody the punk ethos of rebellion and individuality.

Question 67: Which artist is dubbed "The Modfather"?

A Paul Weller

B David Bowie

C Rod Stewart

D Mick Jagger

Question 68: Which song's title translates to "Do It Again" in English?

A La Bamba

B Hasta la Vista

C Bailamos

D Hacerlo Otra Vez

Question 69: Which band's name was inspired by a sculpture in Seattle?

A Soundgarden

B Nirvana

C Pearl Jam

D Foo Fighters

Question 67
A) Paul Weller

Paul Weller, known for his time with The Jam and later The Style Council, is often referred to as "The Modfather" due to his influence on the mod revival movement in Britain. His music consistently reflects the culture and style of the mods, a subculture that first became prominent in the 1960s.

Question 68
D) Hacerlo Otra Vez

"Hacerlo Otra Vez" is Spanish for "Do It Again." While this is not a title of a widely recognized song, it serves as a hypothetical example of how song titles in one language can often be direct translations of those in another, reflecting the universal nature of music.

Question 69
A) Soundgarden

Soundgarden took their name from "A Sound Garden," a wind-channeling sculpture in Seattle that produces musical tones when the wind blows. The band, part of the grunge movement, chose the name to reflect their Seattle roots and their interest in creating a distinct, innovative sound.

Question 70: What instrument is central to Flamenco music?

A	Violin	B	Guitar
C	Piano	D	Harp

Question 71: Which composer is known for the "Hungarian Rhapsodies"?

A	Franz Liszt	B	Johannes Brahms
C	Frédéric Chopin	D	Wolfgang Amadeus Mozart

Question 72: Which artist is known as "The Empress of the Blues"?

A	Etta James	B	Bessie Smith
C	Billie Holiday	D	Ella Fitzgerald

Question 70
B) Guitar

The guitar is central to Flamenco music, a genre originating from Andalusia, Spain. It's known for its emotional intensity, intricate rhythms, and association with dance. The Flamenco guitar, with its distinctive sound and playing technique, is a key element that drives the passionate performances characteristic of this style.

Question 71
A) Franz Liszt

Franz Liszt is famous for his "Hungarian Rhapsodies," a set of 19 piano pieces based on Hungarian folk themes. These works are celebrated for their virtuosity and the way they evoke the spirit of Hungarian gypsy music, showcasing Liszt's innovative and expressive compositional style.

Question 72
B) Bessie Smith

Bessie Smith was dubbed "The Empress of the Blues" for her powerful vocal style and the emotional depth of her performances. She was one of the most popular and influential blues singers of the 1920s and 1930s, with recordings that are considered classics of the genre. Her expressive voice and phrasing have influenced countless artists.

Question 73: What's the name of the dance associated with the tango?

A	Milonga	B	Salsa
C	Waltz	D	Rumba

Question 74: Which song's lyrics include "I shot the sheriff"?

A	Bad Boys	B	Iron Lion Zion
C	No Woman, No Cry	D	I Shot the Sheriff

Question 75: Which artist is known as "The King of Reggae"?

A	Peter Tosh	B	Jimmy Cliff
C	Bob Marley	D	Buju Banton

Question 73
A) Milonga

The milonga is both a style of music and a dance that is closely associated with the tango. Originating in the Rio de la Plata region of Argentina and Uruguay, the milonga is faster-paced than the tango and has a rhythmic, playful character. It's considered a predecessor to the tango and shares many stylistic elements with it.

Question 74
D) I Shot the Sheriff

"I Shot the Sheriff" is a song written by Bob Marley and released in 1973 by The Wailers. The song became famous when Eric Clapton covered it in 1974, and it has since been associated with themes of injustice and defense of personal freedom. The narrative voice in the song claims to have acted in self-defense when shooting the sheriff.

Question 75
C) Bob Marley

Bob Marley is universally known as "The King of Reggae" for his role in popularizing the genre worldwide. His music, which combines elements of reggae, ska, and rocksteady, has had a profound influence on music and culture. His hits like "No Woman, No Cry" and "One Love" remain timeless classics.

Question 76: What's the name of the dance that originated in Harlem in the 1920s?

A	Charleston	B	Tango
C	Salsa	D	Swing

Question 77: Which artist is known as "The Queen of Country"?

A	Dolly Parton	B	Reba McEntire
C	Shania Twain	D	Patsy Cline

Question 78: Which artist's real name is Gordon Sumner?

A	Elton John	B	Sting
C	Bono	D	Moby

Question 76
A) Charleston

The Charleston is a dance that became popular in the 1920s, especially during the Harlem Renaissance. It's characterized by its lively, fast-paced movements and was often danced to ragtime jazz music. The dance captured the exuberant spirit of the Roaring Twenties.

Question 77
A) Dolly Parton

Dolly Parton is often referred to as "The Queen of Country" due to her significant contributions to country music. With a career spanning several decades, she has composed over 3,000 songs, including "Jolene" and "I Will Always Love You." Her distinctive voice and storytelling have made her a beloved icon in the genre.

Question 78
B) Sting

Sting, the lead singer of The Police and a successful solo artist, was born Gordon Sumner. He earned his nickname from the black and yellow striped sweater he wore that looked like a bee. Sting has had a significant impact on rock and pop music with hits like "Roxanne" and "Fields of Gold."

Question 79: Which band's name means "airship" in German?

A. Led Zeppelin
B. Aerosmith
C. Air
D. Jet

Question 80: Which composer is famed for the "Wedding March"?

A. Felix Mendelssohn
B. Johann Pachelbel
C. Richard Wagner
D. Ludwig van Beethoven

Question 81: Which artist is known as "The Man in Black"?

A. Johnny Cash
B. Elvis Presley
C. Bob Dylan
D. Roy Orbison

Question 79
A) Led Zeppelin

Led Zeppelin, an English rock band formed in 1968, took their name from a joke about a "lead balloon" not being able to fly. The name is a play on "lead" (changed to "Led" to avoid mispronunciation) and "Zeppelin," a type of rigid airship named after the German inventor Count Ferdinand von Zeppelin. The band became one of the best-selling music artists in history with their innovative and influential sound.

Question 80
A) Felix Mendelssohn

Felix Mendelssohn composed the "Wedding March" in 1842 as part of his suite for Shakespeare's play "A Midsummer Night's Dream." It has since become one of the most popular pieces of wedding processional music played as the bride walks down the aisle. Mendelssohn's composition has become synonymous with Western wedding ceremonies.

Question 81
A) Johnny Cash

Johnny Cash was known as "The Man in Black" because of his distinctive style of wearing all black during his performances. This look became a symbol of his solidarity with the less fortunate and his stance against social injustices. Cash's deep, calm voice and his narrative-driven songs have left a lasting legacy in country music.

Question 82: Which song features the line "Don't stop believin'"?

(A) Journey - Don't Stop Believin'	(B) Queen - We Are The Champions
(C) Bon Jovi - Livin' on a Prayer	(D) The Beatles - Hey Jude

Question 83: What's the name of the famous jazz club in New York City?

(A) The Blue Note	(B) The Jazz Standard
(C) Birdland	(D) The Village Vanguard

Question 84: Which artist's album is titled "The Velvet Underground & Nico"?

(A) Lou Reed	(B) The Beatles
(C) The Velvet Underground	(D) David Bowie

Question 82
A) Journey - Don't Stop Believin'

"Don't Stop Believin'" is a song by the American rock band Journey, released in 1981. The line "Don't stop believin'" is the song's main refrain and has become an anthem of hope and perseverance. The track gained renewed popularity after being featured in the television series "Glee."

Question 83
C) Birdland

Birdland is a renowned jazz club in New York City, named after the legendary saxophonist Charlie "Bird" Parker. It opened in 1949 and has hosted many famous jazz musicians, becoming a cultural landmark in the jazz world.

Question 84
C) The Velvet Underground

"The Velvet Underground & Nico" is the debut album by The Velvet Underground and features German singer Nico. It was released in 1967 and is notable for its experimental sound and influential artwork by Andy Warhol.

Question 85: Which band's album cover features a prism spectrum?

A. Pink Floyd

B. The Rolling Stones

C. Led Zeppelin

D. The Who

Question 86: Who is known as the "High Priestess of Soul"?

A. Aretha Franklin

B. Nina Simone

C. Billie Holiday

D. Ella Fitzgerald

Question 87: Which song's music video was directed by Michel Gondry?

A. Everlong

B. Around the World

C. Fell in Love with a Girl

D. Bittersweet Symphony

Question 85
A) Pink Floyd

Pink Floyd's album "The Dark Side of the Moon" is famous for its iconic cover art featuring a prism spectrum. The cover was designed by Storm Thorgerson and has become one of the most recognizable album covers in music history.

Question 86
B) Nina Simone

Nina Simone, a singer, pianist, and civil rights activist, was often referred to as the "High Priestess of Soul" for her unique blend of classical, jazz, blues, and gospel music, along with her expressive and emotional performances.

Question 87
B) Around the World

Michel Gondry, known for his inventive visual style, directed the music video for Daft Punk's "Around the World." The video is celebrated for its creative choreography that visually represents the song's layers and beats.

Question 88: Which artist is known for the hit "Fast Car"?

(A)	Tracy Chapman	(B)	Joni Mitchell
(C)	Carole King	(D)	Joan Baez

Question 89: Which artist is known for the song "Your Song"?

(A)	Elton John	(B)	Billy Joel
(C)	Paul McCartney	(D)	Rod Stewart

Question 90: What's the name of the singer known as "Ol' Blue Eyes"?

(A)	Frank Sinatra	(B)	Dean Martin
(C)	Bing Crosby	(D)	Tony Bennett

Question 88
A) Tracy Chapman

"Fast Car" is a song by Tracy Chapman released in 1988. It's known for its storytelling lyrics about a working-class woman's desire to escape her life of poverty. The song was a commercial success and received widespread critical acclaim.

Question 89
A) Elton John

"Your Song" is a famous ballad by Elton John, which appeared on his self-titled second studio album in 1970. The song, with lyrics by Bernie Taupin, was a hit and has been covered by many artists. It remains one of Elton John's most enduring songs.

Question 90
A) Frank Sinatra

Frank Sinatra was affectionately known as "Ol' Blue Eyes" due to his striking blue eyes. He was one of the most popular and influential musical artists of the 20th century, renowned for his smooth voice and timeless classics.

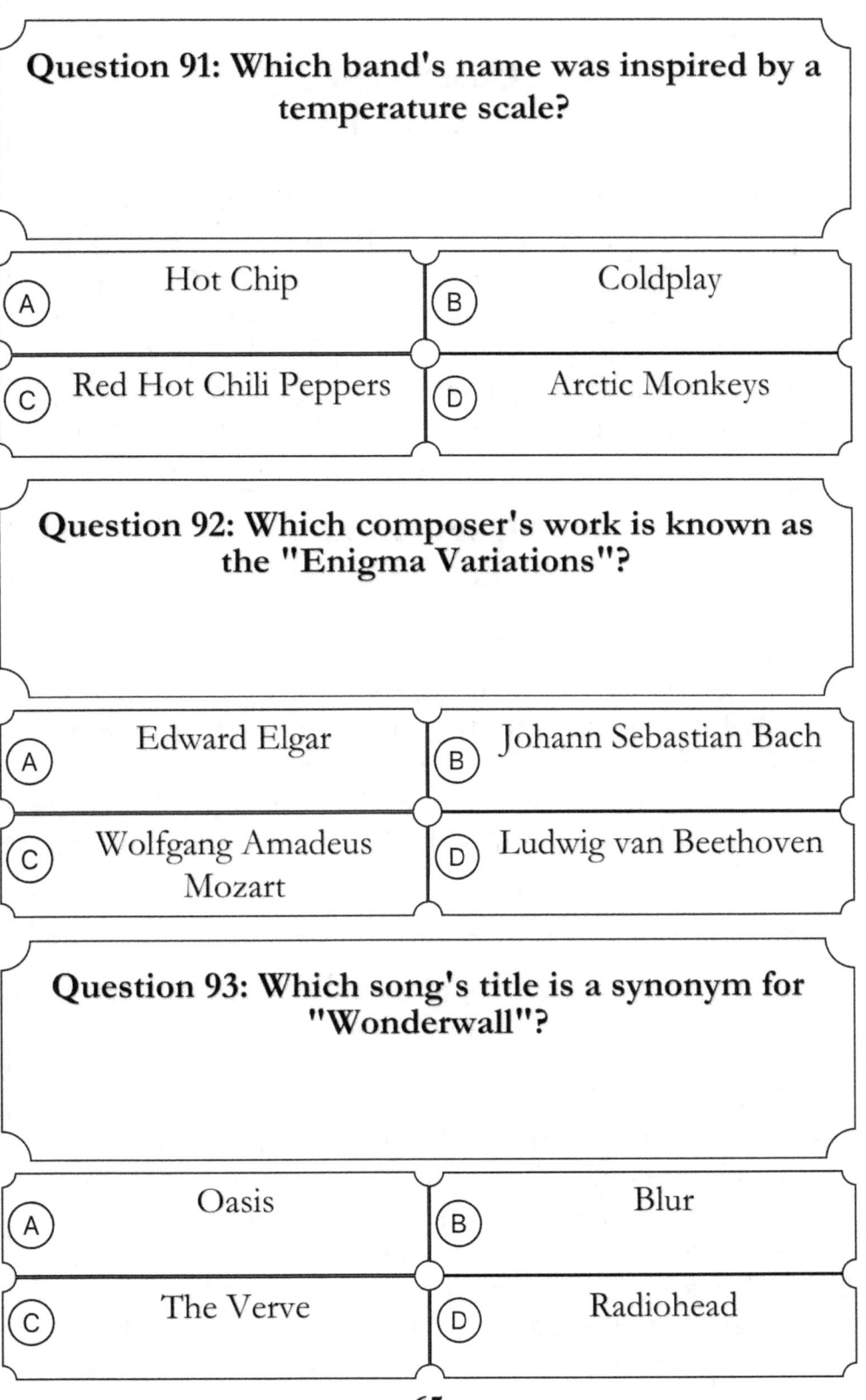

Question 91: Which band's name was inspired by a temperature scale?

A. Hot Chip

B. Coldplay

C. Red Hot Chili Peppers

D. Arctic Monkeys

Question 92: Which composer's work is known as the "Enigma Variations"?

A. Edward Elgar

B. Johann Sebastian Bach

C. Wolfgang Amadeus Mozart

D. Ludwig van Beethoven

Question 93: Which song's title is a synonym for "Wonderwall"?

A. Oasis

B. Blur

C. The Verve

D. Radiohead

Question 91
B) Coldplay

Coldplay's name was inspired by a book of collected poems called "Child's Reflections, Cold Play." The band's original name was Starfish, and they adopted the new name suggested by a friend who had a band also considering the name Coldplay. The term "cold play" is not directly related to a temperature scale, but the name evokes the idea of a cold temperature.

Question 92
A) Edward Elgar

Edward Elgar's "Enigma Variations" is a set of orchestral variations composed between 1898 and 1899. Each variation is a musical sketch of one of Elgar's friends, depicted with affection and humor. The "Enigma" title refers to an undisclosed theme that is not played but is the basis for the variations.

Question 93
A) Oasis

"Wonderwall" is a hit song by the British rock band Oasis, featured on their 1995 album "(What's the Story) Morning Glory?". The song is one of the band's most popular singles and has become an anthem for a generation. The term "wonderwall" means someone who you find yourself thinking about all the time, someone you are completely infatuated with.

Question 94: Which artist is known for the song "Candle in the Wind"?

(A)	Elton John	(B)	Billy Joel
(C)	Bob Dylan	(D)	Paul McCartney

Question 95: Which artist is known for the hit "9 to 5"?

(A)	Dolly Parton	(B)	Reba McEntire
(C)	Shania Twain	(D)	Carrie Underwood

Question 96: What's the title of the song with the lyric "Shake it like a Polaroid picture"?

(A)	Hey Ya!	(B)	Crazy
(C)	Ms. Jackson	(D)	Roses

Question 94
A) Elton John

"Candle in the Wind" is a song by Elton John, originally written in 1973 as a tribute to Marilyn Monroe. It was later re-recorded in 1997 as a tribute to Princess Diana, with the new version becoming the fastest-selling single in UK chart history.

Question 95
A) Dolly Parton

"9 to 5" is a song written and performed by Dolly Parton for the comedy film of the same name. Besides being a hit song, it's also notable for its commentary on the daily grind and empowerment of women in the workplace. The song was released in 1980 and became one of Parton's signature tunes.

Question 96
A) Hey Ya!

The lyric "Shake it like a Polaroid picture" comes from the song "Hey Ya!" by OutKast. The song was released in 2003 and became a huge hit, known for its catchy beat and memorable lyrics. The line became a popular catchphrase and was even addressed by Polaroid as a fun, but not recommended, way to handle their pictures.

Question 97: Which artist is known for the hit "Suspicious Minds"?

A	Elvis Presley	B	Johnny Cash
C	Roy Orbison	D	Jerry Lee Lewis

Question 98: Which band's lead singer is known as "The Lizard King"?

A	The Doors	B	The Beatles
C	The Rolling Stones	D	Led Zeppelin

Question 99: Which artist is known for the hit "Rocket Man"?

A	David Bowie	B	Elton John
C	Rod Stewart	D	Billy Joel

Question 97
A) Elvis Presley

"Suspicious Minds" is one of Elvis Presley's most famous songs, released in 1969. It was a significant comeback hit for Presley, reaching the top of the charts in the US and marking his return to pop music's forefront after a period of movie-making.

Question 98
A) The Doors

"The Lizard King" is a nickname for Jim Morrison, the lead singer of The Doors. The moniker reflects his wild stage persona and poetic lyrics. Morrison is remembered as one of rock music's most iconic and influential frontmen.

Question 99
B) Elton John

"Rocket Man" is a song composed by Elton John and Bernie Taupin and was released in 1972. The song, inspired by a short story by Ray Bradbury, captures the mixed feelings of an astronaut leaving his family to do his job. It's one of Elton John's most beloved songs.

Question 100: Which song is known for the line "Wake me up when September ends"?

A	Green Day	B	Nirvana
C	U2	D	Radiohead

Question 101: Which artist is known for the hit "Tiny Dancer"?

A	Elton John	B	Billy Joel
C	David Bowie	D	Bob Dylan

Question 102: Who is known as the "Father of the Symphony"?

A	A) Ludwig van Beethoven	B	B) Wolfgang Amadeus Mozart
C	C) Joseph Haydn	D	D) Johann Sebastian Bach

Question 100
A) Green Day

"Wake Me Up When September Ends" is a song by Green Day, from their 2004 album "American Idiot." The song was written by lead vocalist Billie Joe Armstrong about his father's death when he was a child. It has become one of the band's most famous ballads.

Question 101
A) Elton John

"Tiny Dancer" is a song by Elton John with lyrics by Bernie Taupin. It appeared on John's 1971 album "Madman Across the Water" and has since been covered by various artists. The song gained renewed popularity after being featured in the film "Almost Famous."

Question 102
C) Joseph Haydn

Joseph Haydn is often referred to as the "Father of the Symphony" due to his significant contributions to the development of the symphonic form. He wrote 104 symphonies and helped establish the structure and style of the symphony that would influence later composers.

Question 103: Which song famously declares "I Will Survive"?

A) A) "Stayin' Alive"

B) B) "I Will Survive"

C) C) "Survivor"

D) D) "Eye of the Tiger"

Question 104: Which band is known for the hit "Under the Bridge"?

A) A) Nirvana

B) B) Red Hot Chili Peppers

C) C) Green Day

D) D) Radiohead

Question 105: What instrument is central to a samba band?

A) A) Guitar

B) B) Drums

C) C) Trumpet

D) D) Piano

Question 103
B) "I Will Survive"

"I Will Survive" is a disco anthem by Gloria Gaynor released in 1978. The song is renowned for its empowering message of strength and perseverance, becoming an enduring symbol of resilience.

Question 104
B) Red Hot Chili Peppers

"Under the Bridge" is a song by the Red Hot Chili Peppers, released in 1992. It became one of their most successful songs, showcasing the band's blend of alternative rock and emotional depth. The song reflects on feelings of loneliness and disconnection.

Question 105
B) Drums

Drums are essential to a samba band, providing the rhythmic foundation that characterizes the genre. The surdo drum, in particular, is known for its deep, resonant beats that drive the samba's tempo.

Question 106: Which composer is known for the "Minute Waltz"?

(A) A) Fr?d?ric Chopin

(B) B) Ludwig van Beethoven

(C) C) Johannes Brahms

(D) D) Franz Liszt

Question 107: Which artist is known for the album "Graceland"?

(A) A) Paul Simon

(B) B) Bruce Springsteen

(C) C) Bob Dylan

(D) D) Eric Clapton

Question 108: Which artist is known for the hit "Livin' on a Prayer"?

(A) A) Bon Jovi

(B) B) Aerosmith

(C) C) Guns N' Roses

(D) D) AC/DC

Question 106
A) Frédéric Chopin

The "Minute Waltz" is the nickname for the "Waltz in D-flat major, Op. 64, No. 1," composed by Frédéric Chopin. It's a piece of solo piano music that is often performed quickly, giving the impression that it lasts only a minute. However, the correct tempo should allow it to run for about two minutes.

Question 107
A) Paul Simon

"Graceland" is the seventh solo studio album by American singer-songwriter Paul Simon. Released in 1986, it won the Grammy Award for Album of the Year in 1987 and is known for its eclectic mixture of musical styles, including pop, a cappella, zydeco, isicathamiya, and mbaqanga.

Question 108
A) Bon Jovi

"Livin' on a Prayer" is a rock anthem by Bon Jovi from their 1986 album "Slippery When Wet." It's one of the band's most well-known songs and has become a staple of rock music. The song tells the story of a working-class couple struggling to make ends meet but remaining hopeful.

Question 109: Who is the lead singer of the band Queen?

A) A) Freddie Mercury

B) B) David Bowie

C) C) Elton John

D) D) Mick Jagger

Question 110: What's the name of the iconic guitar riff in "Smoke on the Water"?

A) A) The Hendrix Riff

B) B) The Slash Riff

C) C) The Blackmore Riff

D) D) The Clapton Riff

Question 111: Which artist is known for the hit "Summer of '69"?

A) A) Bruce Springsteen

B) B) Bryan Adams

C) C) Jon Bon Jovi

D) D) John Mellencamp

Question 109
A) Freddie Mercury

Freddie Mercury was the lead vocalist of the rock band Queen, known for his remarkable vocal range and energetic stage presence. He led the band to international fame with hits like "Bohemian Rhapsody" and "We Are the Champions." Mercury's legacy continues to influence musicians around the world.

Question 110
C) The Blackmore Riff

The iconic guitar riff in Deep Purple's "Smoke on the Water" is often referred to as "The Blackmore Riff," named after the band's guitarist, Ritchie Blackmore. It's one of the most recognizable riffs in rock music history.

Question 111
B) Bryan Adams

"Summer of '69" is one of Bryan Adams' most popular songs, released on his 1984 album "Reckless." The song reminisces about the nostalgic and carefree days of youth and is often celebrated as an iconic summer anthem.

Question 112: Which artist is known for the song "Fire and Rain"?

A) James Taylor

B) Bob Dylan

C) Neil Young

D) Cat Stevens

Question 113: Which band's album is titled "The Joshua Tree"?

A) U2

B) The Rolling Stones

C) Coldplay

D) The Beatles

Question 114: Which artist is known for the song "Piano Man"?

A) Elton John

B) Billy Joel

C) Paul McCartney

D) Bruce Springsteen

Question 112
A) James Taylor

"Fire and Rain" is a folk rock song written and performed by James Taylor. Released in 1970, it became his breakout hit and is known for its reflective lyrics on life's hardships and the search for hope.

Question 113
A) U2*

"The Joshua Tree" is the fifth studio album by Irish rock band U2. Released in 1987, it received critical acclaim and has become one of the world's best-selling albums, with hits like "With or Without You" and "I Still Haven't Found What I'm Looking For." It explores themes of despair, hope, and America's cultural landscape.

Question 114
B) Billy Joel

"Piano Man" is a signature song of Billy Joel, released on his album of the same name in 1973. The song's narrative, which draws on Joel's experiences as a lounge singer, has resonated with audiences for its relatable storytelling and catchy melody.

Question 115: Which band is known for "Stairway to Heaven"?

A) Led Zeppelin

B) Pink Floyd

C) The Eagles

D) The Rolling Stones

Question 116: Which artist is known for the hit "Girls Just Want to Have Fun"?

A) Cyndi Lauper

B) Madonna

C) Whitney Houston

D) Pat Benatar

Question 117: Which artist is known for the song "Respect"?

A) Aretha Franklin

B) Diana Ross

C) Etta James

D) Tina Turner

Question 115
A) Led Zeppelin

"Stairway to Heaven" is a song by the English rock band Led Zeppelin, released in late 1971. It is often regarded as one of the greatest rock songs of all time and is known for its distinctive guitar solo and progressive structure. The song was a staple of Led Zeppelin's live performances and remains a classic in the rock genre.

Question 116
A) Cyndi Lauper

"Girls Just Want to Have Fun" is a song by American artist Cyndi Lauper, released in 1983 as the lead single from her debut album "She's So Unusual." The song became an anthem for female empowerment and is considered one of Lauper's signature songs. It was a major hit and a staple of 1980s pop culture.

Question 117
A) Aretha Franklin

"Respect" is a song made famous by Aretha Franklin after she released her version in 1967. Originally written and recorded by Otis Redding, Franklin's rendition became an anthem for the feminist and civil rights movements and is one of her signature songs. It is widely known for its empowering message and catchy refrain.

Question 118: Which band's album "Hotel California" is a classic?

A) The Eagles

B) Fleetwood Mac

C) The Rolling Stones

D) Pink Floyd

Question 119: Which artist is known for the song "Imagine"?

A) John Lennon

B) Paul McCartney

C) Bob Dylan

D) Elton John

Question 120: Which artist is known for the hit "Sweet Child o' Mine"?

A) Guns N' Roses

B) Aerosmith

C) AC/DC

D) Metallica

Question 118
A) The Eagles

"Hotel California" is the title track from The Eagles' album released in 1976. The song is known for its distinctive guitar solo and cryptic lyrics. The album of the same name is one of the best-selling albums of all time.

Question 119
A) John Lennon

"Imagine" is a song by English rock musician John Lennon from his 1971 album of the same name. The song is one of Lennon's most famous works and is widely regarded as an anthem for peace. Its lyrics encourage listeners to imagine a world without divisions and to live in unity.

Question 120
A) Guns N' Roses

"Sweet Child o' Mine" is a song by American rock band Guns N' Roses, featured on their debut album "Appetite for Destruction" (1987). The song became a huge hit, topping the Billboard Hot 100 chart, and is celebrated for its iconic guitar riff and heartfelt lyrics. It's one of the band's most famous and enduring songs.

Question 121: Which composer is famed for the "Ride of the Valkyries"?

(A) A) Richard Wagner

(B) B) Giuseppe Verdi

(C) C) Johann Strauss II

(D) D) Ludwig van Beethoven

Question 122: Which band's "Sultans of Swing" was a hit?

(A) A) Dire Straits

(B) B) Queen

(C) C) Pink Floyd

(D) D) The Eagles

Question 123: Which artist is known for the hit "Born to Run"?

(A) A) Bruce Springsteen

(B) B) Billy Joel

(C) C) Bob Dylan

(D) D) Tom Petty

Question 121
A) Richard Wagner

"Ride of the Valkyries" is a famous piece from Richard Wagner's opera "Die Walk?re," which is part of his larger work "Der Ring des Nibelungen." The piece is known for its powerful and dramatic music, often associated with the image of valkyries riding into battle. It has become a staple in popular culture.

Question 122
A) Dire Straits

"Sultans of Swing" is a song by British rock band Dire Straits, which first appeared on their self-titled debut album in 1978. The song's distinctive guitar work and unique sound helped establish the band's success and became one of their most well-known tracks. It showcases Mark Knopfler's fingerstyle guitar technique and narrative lyrics.

Question 123
A) Bruce Springsteen

"Born to Run" is a song by American singer-songwriter Bruce Springsteen, and the title track of his 1975 album. The song is a classic rock staple and one of Springsteen's most well-known tracks, celebrated for its energetic sound and sense of youthful aspiration.

Question 124: Which artist is known for the anthem "Fight For Your Right"?

A) A) Beastie Boys

B) B) Nirvana

C) C) Metallica

D) D) Green Day

Question 125: Who is known as the "Father of Bluegrass"?

A) A) Earl Scruggs

B) B) Bill Monroe

C) C) Ralph Stanley

D) D) Lester Flatt

Question 126: Which artist is known as the "Queen of Pop"?

A) A) Madonna

B) B) Lady Gaga

C) C) Beyonc?

D) D) Adele

Question 124
A) Beastie Boys

"Fight For Your Right" is a song by American hip hop group Beastie Boys, released as the fourth single from their debut album "Licensed to Ill" in 1987. The song became an anthem of teenage rebellion and is one of their most recognizable tracks. It parodies the party and rebellious attitude of the time.

Question 125
B) Bill Monroe

Bill Monroe is credited with creating the style of music known as bluegrass, named after his band, the Blue Grass Boys.

Question 126
A) Madonna

Madonna is widely recognized as the "Queen of Pop" for her influence on the music industry during the 1980s, her continual reinvention, and her versatility across various music genres.

Question 127: Which musical features the song "Defying Gravity"?

(A) A) Wicked

(B) B) Rent

(C) C) Cats

(D) D) Hamilton

Question 128: What instrument is iconic to Bluegrass music?

(A) A) Banjo

(B) B) Violin

(C) C) Electric Guitar

(D) D) Piano

Question 129: Which song is famously covered by Johnny Cash?

(A) A) Hurt

(B) B) Imagine

(C) C) Blackbird

(D) D) Hey Jude

Question 127
A) Wicked

"Defying Gravity" is a signature song from the musical "Wicked," which premiered on Broadway in 2003. It's performed by the character Elphaba and symbolizes her decision to live a life unconstrained by others' rules and expectations.

Question 128
A) Banjo

The banjo, with its distinctive twang, is a key instrument in Bluegrass music. This genre, which originated in the Appalachian region of the United States, often features the banjo for its fast-paced and virtuosic playing style.

Question 129
A) Hurt

Johnny Cash's cover of "Hurt," originally by Nine Inch Nails, is renowned for its raw and emotional delivery, which many feel adds depth to the song's themes of regret and redemption.

Question 130: Which artist is famed for the hit "Jolene"?

A) Dolly Parton

B) Patsy Cline

C) Carrie Underwood

D) Shania Twain

Question 131: Which Broadway show tells the story of Alexander Hamilton?

A) Les Mis?rables

B) Hamilton

C) The Phantom of the Opera

D) Chicago

Question 132: Which composer is known for the "1812 Overture"?

A) Tchaikovsky

B) Mozart

C) Beethoven

D) Bach

Question 130
A) Dolly Parton

"Jolene" is one of Dolly Parton's most famous songs, released in 1973. The song is known for its pleading chorus and Parton's expressive storytelling, which have made it a country music classic.

Question 131
B) Hamilton

"Hamilton" is a Broadway musical that blends hip-hop, jazz, R&B, and Broadway styles to tell the story of American Founding Father Alexander Hamilton. It was created by Lin-Manuel Miranda and has received widespread acclaim for its innovative approach to musical theater.

Question 132
A) Tchaikovsky

The "1812 Overture" is a famous orchestral work by Pyotr Ilyich Tchaikovsky. It was written in 1880 to commemorate Russia's defense against Napoleon's invading Grande Arm?e in 1812. The overture is well-known for its inclusion of cannon fire and church bells.

Question 133: What's the signature dance move of Michael Jackson?

A) The Twist

B) The Moonwalk

C) The Macarena

D) Gangnam Style

Question 134: Which artist is known for the hit "I Walk the Line"?

A) Johnny Cash

B) Elvis Presley

C) Bob Dylan

D) Bruce Springsteen

Question 135: Which band is known for the album "American Idiot"?

A) Green Day

B) Blink-182

C) The Offspring

D) Sum 41

Question 133
B) The Moonwalk

Michael Jackson's signature dance move, the Moonwalk, became famous after he performed it during the song "Billie Jean" on a 1983 television special. It involves sliding the foot backwards while keeping the illusion of walking forwards.

Question 134
A) Johnny Cash

"I Walk the Line" is a classic song by Johnny Cash, released in 1956. It's one of his most famous works, known for its unique rhythm and deep, distinctive vocals. The song reflects Cash's commitment to stay faithful to his first wife, Vivian Liberto.

Question 135
A) Green Day

"American Idiot" is a Grammy Award-winning album by the punk rock band Green Day, released in 2004. It's a concept album that critiques the state of the United States at the time and is known for its politically charged lyrics.

Question 136: What's the name of the dance where dancers form a line?

A) Tango

B) Waltz

C) Conga

D) Salsa

Question 137: Which artist is known for the song "Firework"?

A) Katy Perry

B) Taylor Swift

C) Rihanna

D) Ariana Grande

Question 138: Which composer is known for "The Four Seasons"?

A) Vivaldi

B) Bach

C) Handel

D) Mozart

Question 136
C) Conga

The Conga is a dance of Afro-Cuban origin where dancers form a long, single-file line. Typically, it's performed at parties, weddings, and other festive events, with participants moving rhythmically in a snake-like formation.

Question 137
A) Katy Perry

"Firework" is a hit song by Katy Perry from her album "Teenage Dream," released in 2010. The song is an empowerment anthem, encouraging listeners to embrace their uniqueness and shine brightly.

Question 138
A) Vivaldi

Antonio Vivaldi, an Italian Baroque composer, is famous for "The Four Seasons," a group of four violin concerti, each representing a season. It's celebrated for its vivid imagery of nature and its innovative orchestration.

Question 139: Which artist's album "Back to Black" won five Grammy Awards?

A	A) Amy Winehouse	B	B) Adele
C	C) Norah Jones	D	D) Lauryn Hill

Question 140: Which artist is known for the hit "Say My Name"?

A	A) Destiny's Child	B	B) TLC
C	C) Spice Girls	D	D) No Doubt

Question 141: Which show features the song "The Phantom of the Opera"?

A	A) Cats	B	B) Les Mis?rables
C	C) The Phantom of the Opera	D	D) Rent

Question 139
A) Amy Winehouse

Amy Winehouse's "Back to Black" album, released in 2006, received critical acclaim and won five Grammy Awards, including Best Pop Vocal Album and Record of the Year for the song "Rehab." It's known for its blend of soul, jazz, and R&B.

Question 140
A) Destiny's Child

"Say My Name" is one of Destiny's Child's most iconic songs, released in 1999. It won the Best R&B Performance by a Duo or Group with Vocals and Best R&B Song at the 43rd Annual Grammy Awards.

Question 141
C) The Phantom of the Opera

"The Phantom of the Opera" is the title song from the musical of the same name, composed by Andrew Lloyd Webber. It's one of Broadway's longest-running shows and is known for its dramatic and romantic score.

Question 142: Who is known as the "Father of Country Music"?

A) Hank Williams

B) Johnny Cash

C) Jimmie Rodgers

D) George Jones

Question 143: Which song is considered the anthem of country music?

A) Friends in Low Places

B) The Dance

C) I Walk the Line

D) Crazy

Question 144: Which opera features the "Queen of the Night" aria?

A) Carmen

B) The Magic Flute

C) La Traviata

D) Rigoletto

Question 142
C) Jimmie Rodgers

Jimmie Rodgers is often referred to as the "Father of Country Music" due to his significant influence on the genre. His blend of traditional folk, blues, and yodeling set the foundation for modern country music.

Question 143
A) Friends in Low Places

"Friends in Low Places" by Garth Brooks is often hailed as an anthem of country music. Released in 1990, it's known for its relatable lyrics and sing-along chorus, embodying the spirit of country music's camaraderie and resilience.

Question 144
B) The Magic Flute

The "Queen of the Night" aria is a famous coloratura soprano piece from Mozart's opera "The Magic Flute." It's known for its demanding vocal range and is a highlight of the opera, showcasing the Queen's fury and vocal prowess.

Question 145: Which artist is credited with popularizing the "crooning" style?

A) Frank Sinatra

B) Bing Crosby

C) Dean Martin

D) Tony Bennett

Question 146: Which instrument is known for its use in Fado music?

A) Guitarra Portuguesa

B) Violin

C) Harp

D) Accordion

Question 147: Which artist is known for the hit "Rolling in the Deep"?

A) Adele

B) Beyonc?

C) Sam Smith

D) Ed Sheeran

Question 145
B) Bing Crosby

Bing Crosby is widely regarded as the pioneer of the "crooning" style, a smooth, relaxed way of singing that became popular in the 1930s. His warm baritone voice and

Question 146
A) Guitarra Portuguesa

The Guitarra Portuguesa, a Portuguese guitar, is a key instrument in Fado music, a genre that originated in Portugal. It's known for its distinctive sound and is often used to convey the genre's melancholic and soulful melodies.

Question 147
A) Adele

"Rolling in the Deep" is a song by the English singer Adele from her second studio album, "21." Released in 2010, it became one of the best-selling singles of all time and won the Grammy Award for Record of the Year and Song of the Year. The song's powerful vocals and soulful rhythm helped solidify Adele's status as a global superstar.

Question 148: Which band's album is titled "Abbey Road"?

A) The Beatles

B) The Rolling Stones

C) Pink Floyd

D) Queen

Question 149: Who is known as the "Father of Bluegrass"?

A. Earl Scruggs

B. Bill Monroe

C. Ralph Stanley

D. Lester Flatt

Question 150: Which genre is characterized by "shredding" guitar solos?

A) Blues

B) Jazz

C) Heavy Metal

D) Classical

Question 148
A) The Beatles

"Abbey Road" is a critically acclaimed album by The Beatles, released in 1969. It's renowned for its innovative production and is famous for its iconic cover photo featuring the band crossing a zebra crossing outside Abbey Road Studios.

Question 149
B) Bill Monroe

Bill Monroe is credited with creating the style of music known as bluegrass, named after his band, the Blue Grass Boys.

Question 150
C) Heavy Metal

"Shredding" refers to a virtuosic guitar solo playing style featuring fast runs and advanced techniques. It's most commonly associated with the Heavy Metal genre, where it showcases the guitarist's skill and speed.

Afterword

As the final notes of this musical trivia journey fade into a satisfying silence, I want to take a moment to express my heartfelt gratitude to you, the reader. Your engagement and enthusiasm have transformed what could have been mere words on a page into a lively symphony of shared knowledge and joy.

This book was composed with the hope of not only testing your musical acumen but also of reigniting a passion for the stories, the personalities, and the cultural movements that have shaped the soundtrack of our lives. If you've found yourself humming a forgotten melody or rediscovering a classic album, then this book has fulfilled its purpose.

Your participation in this trivia is a testament to the universal language of music—a language that transcends borders, connects hearts, and enriches souls. As you close this book, may the echoes of the questions and answers inspire you to continue exploring the vast and beautiful world of music.

If this book has struck a chord with you, consider sharing your experience with others. Your reviews and recommendations are the ripples that can turn this solitary activity into a chorus of communal discovery.

Thank you for playing your part in this melody. Until our next musical encounter, keep the rhythm alive and the harmony flowing.

With appreciation and musical regards,
Leon Simonds